INTERMITTENT

FASTING

I0425812

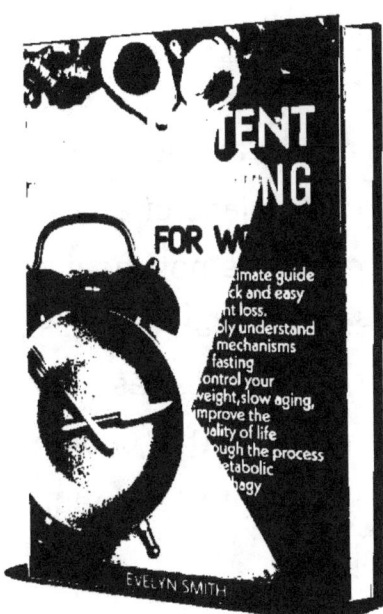 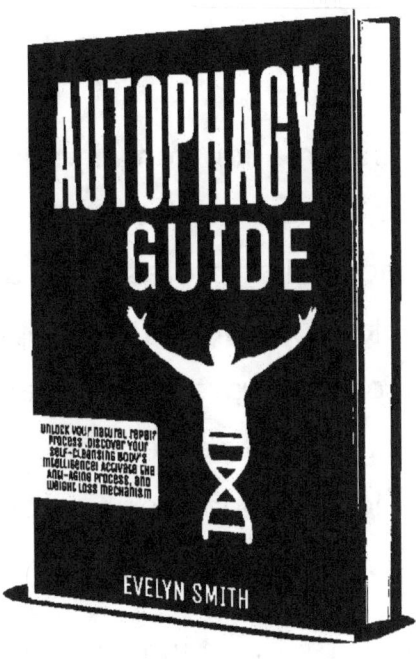

INTERMITTENTFASTING FOR WOMEN +
AUTOPHAGY GUIDE

2 ESSENTIAL TOOLS FOR YOUR HEALTH

Evelyn Smith

Legal & Disclaimer

The information contained in this book and its contents is not designed to replace or take the place of any form of medical or professional advice; and is not meant to replace the need for independent medical, financial, legal or other professional advice or services, as may be required. The content and information in this book has been provided for educational and entertainment purposes only.

The content and information contained in this book has been compiled from sources deemed reliable, and it is accurate to the best of the Author's knowledge, information and belief. However, the Author cannot guarantee its accuracy and validity and cannot be held liable for any errors and/or omissions. Further, changes are periodically made to this book as and when needed. Where appropriate and/or necessary, you must consult a professional (including but not limited to your doctor, attorney, financial advisor or such other professional advisor) before using any of the suggested remedies, techniques, or information in this book.

Upon using the contents and information contained in this book, you agree to hold harmless the Author from and against any damages, costs, and expenses, including any legal fees potentially resulting from the application of any of the information provided by this book. This disclaimer applies to any loss, damages or injury caused by the use and application, whether directly or indirectly, of any advice or information presented, whether for breach of contract, tort, negligence, personal injury, criminal intent, or under any other cause of action.

You agree to accept all risks of using the information presented inside this book.

You agree that by continuing to read this book, where appropriate and/or necessary, you shall consult a professional (including but not limited to your doctor, attorney, or financial advisor or such other advisor as needed) before using any of the suggested remedies, techniques, or information in this book

Table of Contents

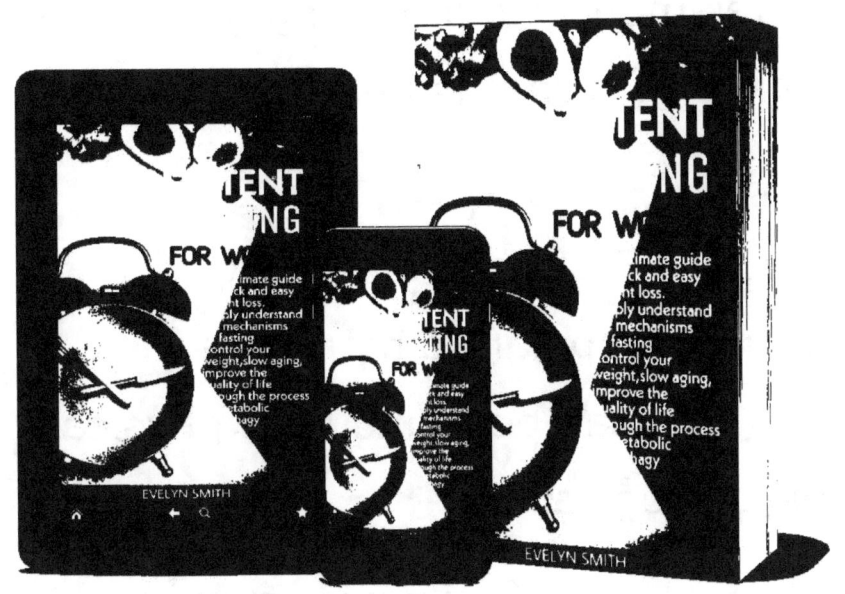

INTERMITTENT FASTING FOR WOMEN introduction

A new diet has been introduced for some time: the intermittent fasting diet (also called Intermittent Fasting)

In reality, as we will see better in the course of the article, intermittent fasting is not a real diet but a food program that alternates moments of fasting with intervals on which it is instead allowed to feed.

Intermittent Fasting is becoming increasingly popular as many are the benefits that can be found both physically and psychologically.

Moreover, this type of power supply is also very convenient and practical and adapts very well to our increasingly rapid and frenetic lifestyle.

So if your goal is to lose the extra pounds, then you are in the right place at the right time, because today I will reveal all the details of a truly effective food program proven by various nutritionists.

If you want to learn more then read on below and you will discover the multiple positive effects that you can achieve with the Intermittent Fasting Diet

How does intermittent fasting work?
Let's start with the basics ...

What exactly is the diet called "Intermittent Fasting"?

It is a dietary approach in which you will have to enter within the day (or week, depending on the choice you will make when you set the strategic plan), a time of minimum 12-16 hours of fasting, such as to affect the overall caloric balance and hormonal metabolism.

In practice there are two phases:

• a fasting phase called fast, lasting several hours (usually 12 to 20 hours) in which you will not have to introduce any food, except for beverages, such as water, tea, bitter coffee or sugar-free herbal teas

• a phase called fed where you can eat regularly

That's all? That's all.

The Intermittent Fasting is in fact very simple. And that's why it works very well! Soon I'll also explain why.

But first I want to give you some more details.

In fact, there are several methods of intermittent fasting:

1. Intermittent Fasting 16/8: this scheme divides the day into two parts, that is, 8 hours you eat (Fed) and 16 hours of fast (Fast). An example of application is this: skip breakfast and consume the first meal at noon and then don't eat until 20:00.

2. Every other day (5: 2): for two days a week the calorie intake must be reduced to 500-600 calories, while for the rest of the week you can eat what you want. Of course for this type of diet, the days where the calorie intake is reduced must not be consecutive.

3. Eat stop eat: eat once or twice a week from the evening of the day before until dinner the next day.

As you can see, even in this case they are all extremely simple and allow great flexibility

Intermittent Fasting May Affect Men and Women Differently

There is some evidence that intermittent fasting may not be as beneficial for some women as it is for men.

One study showed that blood sugar control actually worsened in women after three weeks of intermittent fasting, which was not the case in men.

There are also many anecdotal stories of women who have experienced changes to their menstrual cycles after starting intermittent fasting.

Such shifts occur because female bodies are extremely sensitive to calorie restriction.

When calorie intake is low — such as from fasting for too long or too frequently — a small part of the brain called the hypothalamus is affected.

This can disrupt the secretion of gonadotropin-releasing hormone (GnRH), a hormone that helps release two reproductive hormones: luteinizing hormone (LH) and follicle stimulating hormone (FSH).

When these hormones cannot communicate with the ovaries, you run the risk of irregular periods, infertility, poor bone health and other health effects.

Although there are no comparable human studies, tests in rats have shown that 3–6 months of alternate-day fasting caused a reduction in ovary size and irregular reproductive cycles in female rats .

For these reasons, women should consider a modified approach to intermittent fasting, such as shorter fasting periods and fewer fasting days.

Intermittent fasting to lose weight:

Obviously when we talk about food the first thought goes to the weight and the balance. And therefore to the question: with intermittent fasting is it possible to lose weight?

Absolutely yes! But not only.

If you want to achieve one or all of these three goals:

- Lose weight

- correct various health problems

- live longer

... then this diet is just for you!

In fact it is a great expedient to combine the need to reduce caloric intake and at the same time lighten the effort to give up calories in a natural way.

Having followed many people who wanted to lose weight and who had tried the most varied diets before intermittent fasting, I can say from experience that this methodology is one of those that guarantees the best results.

Not only for the quantity of kilograms lost but above all for the quality of weight loss (very well balanced between lean mass and fat mass) and for ease of weight maintenance once you reach your goal?

How is it possible?

I'll explain why.

There are many people who undertake a diet but very few carry it out. Why do you think? I'll tell you: because it's difficult to give up your favorite foods and because you can't resist the urge to go hungry.

With intermittent fasting, however, both these seemingly insurmountable obstacles are circumvented.

Fasting in fact puts the body in the condition of not having enough energy from food and therefore having to take it from internal reserves (leading to weight loss). Without, however, causing that hunger that we usually feel when we are on a low-calorie diet (reduced in calories).

It seems paradoxical but it is so. Where is the trick?

In the limited duration of fasting.

A prolonged fast in fact demotivates the person, besides putting in place a whole series of compensations from our body, some of which absolutely to be avoided.

While instead fasting only for a limited time makes this practice much easier, because fasting is relatively short and consequently is more bearable.

Other benefits of intermittent fasting

Intermittent Fasting is not only useful for weight loss ... it is a real system to stay healthy for a long time.

In fact, fasting is one of the most powerful means of purifying the body.

When our body is not busy processing food all the time it can devote itself to other activities, such as "cleaning" our body of waste and making many metabolic processes more efficient.

Not to mention the hormonal impact of Intermittent Fasting

Fasting allows us to make our cells more resistant to insulin, promoting protection from important metabolic disorders such as diabetes and the metabolic syndrome.

And finally, during the periods of short fasting, important increases in the production of Growth Hormone have been detected, an important mediator of cell regeneration, useful not only for sportsmen but more generally for all people who wish to slow down the aging process.

How can you guess intermittent fasting is not one of the usual diets that promise miracles in a few weeks.

This is a type of diet that aims to speed up the metabolism and help you lose weight faster by improving cardiovascular health and the immune system in general.

The concept on which it is born is to temporarily disrupt your body and your metabolism, changing the way you usually work your target and forcing it to "wake up" with interesting 360 ° benefits

If you want to undertake this type of diet you will not only lose the extra pounds, but your immune system will become much more resistant to disease.

Many people who have considered this type of diet have felt better physically, and during that time, they felt more energy

Health Benefits of Intermittent Fasting for Women

Intermittent fasting not only benefits your waistline but may also lower your risk of developing a number of chronic diseases.

Heart Health

Heart disease is the leading cause of death worldwide .

High blood pressure, high LDL cholesterol and high triglyceride concentrations are some of the leading risk factors for the development of heart disease.

One study in 16 obese men and women showed intermittent fasting lowered blood pressure by 6% in just eight weeks.

The same study also found that intermittent fasting lowered LDL cholesterol by 25% and triglycerides by 32% .

However, the evidence for the link between intermittent fasting and improved LDL cholesterol and triglyceride levels is not consistent.

A study in 40 normal-weight people found that four weeks of intermittent fasting during the Islamic holiday of Ramadan did not result in a reduction in LDL cholesterol or triglycerides.

Higher-quality studies with more robust methods are needed before researchers can fully understand the effects of intermittent fasting on heart health.

Diabetes

Intermittent fasting may also effectively help manage and reduce your risk of developing diabetes.

Similar to continuous calorie restriction, intermittent fasting appears to reduce some of the risk factors for diabetes.

It does so mainly by lowering insulin levels and reducing insulin resistance.

In a randomized controlled study of more than 100 overweight or obese women, six months of intermittent fasting reduced insulin levels by 29% and insulin resistance by 19%. Blood sugar levels remained the same.

What's more, 8–12 weeks of intermittent fasting has been shown to lower insulin levels by 20–31% and blood sugar levels by 3–6% in individuals with pre-diabetes, a condition in which blood sugar levels are elevated but not high enough to diagnose diabetes .

However, intermittent fasting may not be as beneficial for women as it is for men in terms of blood sugar.

A small study found that blood sugar control worsened for women after 22 days of alternate-day fasting, while there was no adverse effect on blood sugar for men

.

Despite this side effect, the reduction in insulin and insulin resistance would still likely reduce the risk of diabetes, particularly for individuals with pre-diabetes.

Weight Loss

Intermittent fasting can be a simple and effective way to lose weight when done properly, as regular short-term fasts can help you consume fewer calories and shed pounds.

A number of studies suggest that intermittent fasting is as effective as traditional calorie-restricted diets for short-term weight loss .

A 2018 review of studies in overweight adults found intermittent fasting led to an average weight loss of 15 lbs (6.8 kg) over the course of 3–12 months.

Another review showed intermittent fasting reduced body weight by 3–8% in overweight or obese adults over a period of 3–24 weeks. The review also found that participants reduced their waist circumference by 3–7% over the same period .

It should be noted that the long-term effects of intermittent fasting on weight loss for women remain to be seen.

In the short term, intermittent fasting seems to aid in weight loss. However, the amount you lose will likely depend on the number of calories you consume during non-fasting periods and how long you adhere to the lifestyle.

It May Help You Eat Less

Switching to intermittent fasting may naturally help you eat less.

One study found that young men ate 650 fewer calories per day when their food intake was restricted to a four-hour window .

Another study in 24 healthy men and women looked at the effects of a long, 36-hour fast on eating habits. Despite consuming extra calories on the post-fast day, participants dropped their total calorie balance by 1,900 calories, a significant reduction .

Other Health Benefits

A number of human and animal studies suggest that intermittent fasting may also yield other health benefits.

Reduced inflammation: Some studies show that intermittent fasting can reduce key markers of inflammation. Chronic inflammation can lead to weight gain and various health problems .

Improved psychological well-being: One study found that eight weeks of intermittent fasting decreased depression and binge eating behaviors while improving body image in obese adults .

Increased longevity: Intermittent fasting has been shown to extend lifespan in rats and mice by 33–83%. The effects on longevity in humans is yet to be determined .

Preserve muscle mass: Intermittent fasting appears to be more effective at retaining muscle mass compared to continuous calorie restriction. Higher muscle mass helps you burn more calories, even at rest.

Specifically, the health benefits of intermittent fasting for women need to be studied more extensively in well-designed human studies before any conclusions can be drawn .

Frequently Asked Questions

Here are answers to the most common questions about intermittent fasting.

1. Can I Drink Liquids During the Fast?

Yes. Water, coffee, tea and other non-caloric beverages are fine. Do not add sugar to your coffee. Small amounts of milk or cream may be okay.

Coffee can be particularly beneficial during a fast, as it can blunt hunger.

2. Isn't It Unhealthy to Skip Breakfast?

No. The problem is that most stereotypical breakfast skippers have unhealthy lifestyles. If you make sure to eat healthy food for the rest of the day then the practice is perfectly healthy.

3. Can I Take Supplements While Fasting?

Yes. However, keep in mind that some supplements like fat-soluble vitamins may work better when taken with meals.

4. Can I Work out While Fasted?

Yes, fasted workouts are fine. Some people recommend taking branched-chain amino acids (BCAAs) before a fasted workout.

You can find many BCAA products on Amazon.

5. Will Fasting Cause Muscle Loss?

All weight loss methods can cause muscle loss, which is why it's important to lift weights and keep your protein intake high. One study showed that intermittent fasting causes less muscle loss than regular calorie restriction (16Trusted Source).

6. Will Fasting Slow Down My Metabolism?

No. Studies show that short-term fasts actually boost metabolism (14Trusted Source, 15Trusted Source). However, longer fasts of 3 or more days can suppress metabolism (36Trusted Source).

7. Should Kids Fast?

Allowing your child to fast is probably a bad idea.

Does intermittent fasting work?

We hear about fasting since ancient times. Many peoples of the world have practiced fasting for purifying, healthy and religious reasons.

And in fact the origins of fasting are lost in the mists of time.

Many even claim that fasting is the "normal mode of functioning of the human being". In fact, if you think about it, over the millennia there has never been such availability of food as it is today.

Therefore the man of the past, for hundreds of thousands of years, has always fasted.

He almost always fasted, at least until the hunters of the tribe could not hunt some big animal, thus giving the possibility to all the various families to take refreshment and "fill up with food"

This phenomenon has happened for a very long time. It is practically inherent in our DNA.

In a world characterized by scarcity of food, the interval of fasting periods more or less long and periods of "binge eating" is practically normal.

This is exactly why intermittent fasting works.

In fact, with the intermittent fasting diet, you introduce nutrients in a cyclic way (the two phases that alternate) and this is a good thing since this regime respects the physiology of the human body.

So, when asked, intermittent fasting works, the answer is certainly yes.

This is a powerful tool that, once you understand how it works, will help you lose excess weight, maintain a healthy weight, live longer and get rid of many diseases.

Types of Intermittent Fasting

The following are the most popular examples of intermittent fasting and can be adapted as needed. In the Intermittent Fasting Guide you will find an in-depth look at each of the types of fasting listed, which can be associated with a sport.

Diet LeanGains or Intermittent Fasting 16: 8

The LeanGains diet or intermittent fasting 16: 8 provides a feeding window - feeding window - of 8 hours followed by 16 hours of fasting. In the most basic version, we essentially skip breakfast.

Intermittent Fasting 18: 6

Similar to the LeanGains diet. Here the feeding window is 6 hours and fasting for 8 hours.

Fast or 5: 2 diet

For 5 days a week we eat in a classic way. In the remaining two, around 500 calories are consumed.

Warrior Diet or Warrior Diet

The feeding window is 4 hours, usually for dinner. In the rest of the day you can choose to consume fresh vegetables and light fruit.

Alternating Fasting or Alternating-day Fasting

A day of fasting alternates with a day when food is consumed. The day you eat you can choose to do it all day or in a specific feeding window.

OMAD diet

The OMAD diet - One Meal A Day - includes a feeding window of 1 hour a day and 23 hours of fasting. In practice, a full meal a day.

Complete fasting

Once a week or when you want to fast for a whole day. On other days you can choose whether to follow intermittent fasting or not. It is also possible to fast more

lunch, as for example for 5 days.

Best Types of Intermittent Fasting for Women

When it comes to dieting, there is no one-size-fits-all approach. This also applies to intermittent fasting.

Generally speaking, women should take a more relaxed approach to fasting than men.

This may include shorter fasting periods, fewer fasting days and/or consuming a small number of calories on the fasting days.

Here are some of the best types of intermittent fasting for women

Crescendo Method: Fasting 12–16 hours for two to three days a week. Fasting days should be nonconsecutive and spaced evenly across the week (for example, Monday, Wednesday and Friday).

Eat-stop-eat (also called the 24-hour protocol): A 24-hour full fast once or twice a week (maximum of two times a week for women). Start with 14–16 hour fasts and gradually build up.

The 5:2 Diet (also called "The Fast Diet"): Restrict calories to 25% of your usual intake (about 500 calories) for two days a week and eat "normally" the other five days. Allow one day between fasting days.

Modified Alternate-Day Fasting: Fasting every other day but eating "normally" on non-fasting days. You are allowed to consume 20–25% of your usual calorie intake (about 500 calories) on a fasting day.

The 16/8 Method (also called the "Leangains method"): Fasting for 16 hours a day and eating all calories within an eight-hour window. Women are advised to start with 14-hour fasts and eventually build up to 16 hours.

Whichever you choose, it is still important to eat well during the non-fasting periods. If you eat a large amount of unhealthy, calorie-dense foods during the non-fasting periods, you may not experience the same weight loss and health benefits.

At the end of the day, the best approach is one that you can tolerate and sustain in the long-term, and which does not result in any negative health consequences.

Easier fasting

Yes, because in reality very few people are endowed with the momentum and willpower needed to face a fast that can last up to several days.

Hence the desire for a simpler and more feasible alternative ...

Fasting is one of the most powerful means of resetting unbalanced biochemistry and optimizing conditions that can lead to life extension. But for many people it is difficult to implement, especially for two reasons ...

How is intermittent fasting easier?

Two of the main reasons why prolonged fasting is difficult to implement are the following.

First of all it would be appropriate to take the time dedicated to a prolonged depurative ritual. Then it is advised to set up also the best conditions to operate a fast (to be followed by a nutritionist or by the doctor, to be able to remain focused on this goal, etc.) given the effort required to complete it (it is useless to deny it).

In short, putting a prolonged fasting into practice decidedly difficult makes it difficult if not impossible for many people to approach this healthy practice.

At most, many well-intentioned people simply read something about fasting, try, then get upset and give up and don't try anymore ...

But thanks to intermittent fasting the practice of abstaining from food (and calories in general) becomes decidedly easier for everyone to implement.

Also because unlike prolonged fasting, which may require an interruption of the most demanding activities, intermittent fasting takes advantage of daily tasks

Distract yourself and fast

In what sense does it "take advantage of daily commitments"? pulling a single day without eating can be even easier to bear if you are immersed in your usual activities in the meantime.

So with intermittent fasting there is no need to change anything of one's daily activity rituals. Indeed these can just distract the mind from the thought of food.

A brief workout such as functional training or 30-45 minute yoga on the day of this short fast would even be recommended.

Finally, with a minimum of good will, anyone can FAST and gain health and fitness without necessarily having the mental strength of a fakir.

Another grandiose element of intermittent fasting that facilitates its implementation concerns the fact that it is relatively elastic in its duration. That is, the time to devote to fasting is relatively short, therefore bearable

Characteristics of intermittent fasting

Intermittent fasting is an extremely natural way of eating.

During its evolution, the complex and refined metabolism of the human being was forged by an innumerable series of intermittent fasts, not binge eating!

If you think about the difficulty of getting nourishment in nature you can guess that the body has all the means to survive days and days with little or nothing.

Our body is perfectly designed to pass through more or less long periods of absence of food. Not only can it do but it is also a prerogative for its optimal functioning.

It is more normal for us to fast intermittently than to eat 3 or 4 times a day. That is to say, the unhealthy deviation consists precisely in feeding too much, so the remedy is to return to the natural rhythms of intermittent fasting.

Religious fasting

Furthermore, in the course of our most recent evolution, intermittent fasting has continued to be present and widespread for religious reasons. In many different religions and rituals around the world the need has always been felt to devote periods of time to abstaining from food.

Voluntary abstention from food is a form of self-discipline that increases the perception of control that our mind can have on the body. Unleashed desires often cause unhappiness that lasts long after the brief enjoyment of their immediate satisfaction

A certain inner solidity due to the fact of "taking back the bridles" of our behavior is associated with greater happiness. This is probably why religions often prescribe programmed food waivers.

Certainly today numerous researches confirm that the metabolic rest that can be implemented with intermittent fasting is one of the most effective and easy to implement ways to get better and live longer

4 ways in which intermittent fasting changes metabolism.

When you stop taking calories for enough time in your body, certain cellular and molecular changes occur ...

1) Activation of autophagy

One of the most important events taking place in a fasting organism is autophagy[1,2]. The intelligence of the body under the stimulus of lack of energy from food sources (during fasting) begins to exploit damaged cells and molecules to feed themselves.

The body thus begins to sustain itself thanks to the use of some of its components now aged and therefore to be replaced. Autophagy in this way expresses two benefits in one: it supplies new energy to the body and at the same time eliminates certain parts that are now dysfunctional.

... AND CELL REGENERATION

Following the elimination of damaged components the body is induced to synthesize new ones. The newly generated components (cells, proteins, etc.) will be healthier than the previous ones because they are just "churned out" by the body's biosynthetic system.

Whenever this cycle of elimination and regeneration occurs, the body is partly renewed and renewed, prolonging its longevity potential.

Not bad...

With a simple short (intermittent) fast the body renews itself.

We had already encountered this process in the practice of the fasting diet. Certainly, however, this last approach is definitely more challenging because it lasts 5 days. On the contrary, an intermittent fasting lasts only from 16 to 24 hours (including the hours of natural night fasting).

2) Synthesis of the GH hormone

GH is the acronym of Growth Hormone, that is growth hormone.

This hormone simultaneously activates the development of muscle mass and the loss of body fat3. Two important benefits for maintaining a lean and healthy body.

The body tends to produce less GH over the years during the aging process. Fasting makes it possible to give a new boost to the production of this important hormone4,5 in a completely natural way

3)Profilo insulinico

With intermittent fasting the insulin sensitivity improves and consequently the average insulin levels are lowered. This allows easier access to the use of deposited fat reserves

3) Insulin profile

During an intermittent fasting practice several protective action genes are activated. In particular, protective genes are activated against different pathologies7 and genes closely involved in the mechanisms of longevity

The 5 Benefits of Intermittent Fasting # 1) Weight Loss

Intermittent fasting is truly a powerful way to reduce excess fat. Its action on specific hormones such as GH, insulin and noradrenaline makes it an effective tool to reduce abdominal inflammatory fat (see article on belly fat).

Moreover, even the calorie reduction in the strict sense that occurs during intermittent fasting contributes to weight

2) Anti-inflammatory effect

Several studies show that fasting reduces the inflammatory state of the body9,10.

This leads to a consequent benefit against numerous chronic degenerative pathologies that develop starting from a chronic inflammatory condition.

3) Heart health

A series of benefits of intermittent fasting linked to heart health 11 makes it particularly suitable for maintaining the cardiovascular system in perfect condition.

Specifically, intermittent fasting can reduce inflammation, blood sugars (improve insulin sensitivity), triglycerides and "bad" LDL cholesterol. All this produces a synergy that promotes the health of the heart and arteries

#4) Antitumor protection

Several studies show a correlation between intermittent fasting and special protection against cancer cells12,13. By now it is becoming increasingly clear how reducing the quantity and frequency of meals can protect better than any other defense against the development of "mad cells"

#5) Maintenance and optimization of brain and nerve functions

This benefit of intermittent fasting is associated with its general anti-aging effect but is also expressed markedly in relation to neurons.

Some studies show that intermittently fasting stimulates the processes of nerve regeneration15 (postnatal neurogenesis). It also protects against neurodegenerative diseases16.17 and against Alzheimer's disease18.

AND AN ADDITIONAL BENEFIT ...

To this list of 5 points that you have just seen, I would also add another very useful side benefit ... increase your willpower. Willpower is like a muscle that increases its power with training.

More willpower means greater self-control in our lives. A wise and non-violent self-control helps to direct our lives constructively and thus leads us to a greater good

How intermittent fasting works

Intermittent fasting is nothing exotic ... who knows how many times you have already put it into practice without knowing it.

Maybe because of the haste and the little time available you missed the breakfast arriving until lunchtime without taking calories of any kind. This is a classic example of intermittent "unconscious" fasting.

One of the most beautiful things that make intermittent fasting easy to follow even for the less "aggressive" is that you can take advantage of the hours of sleep. The hours of sleep are counted in the minimum 16 hours of fasting.

To begin the practice of intermittent fasting you can easily dine and then no longer touch food or calories of any kind until lunchtime the next day.

Indeed...

The time range for caloric abstention is from 16 to 24 hours (uninterrupted). A short time, especially if you think that in this count the hours of sleep are already included.

Intermittent fasting easy version

Duration: 16 hours (including overnight fasting).

Mode: starts with dinner, say at 8.00pm. For example, if you finish dinner at 20:30. From that moment on, no food is touched until 12:30 on the following day.

Intermittent fasting Intermediate version

Of course you can decide to make any intermediate version between 16-24 hours. For example, let's say you want to do 18 hours of fasting and finish dinner at

8.30pm ... in this case, don't touch food until 2.30pm the following day.

Intermittent fasting difficult version

Duration: 24 hours (including overnight fasting)

Mode: starts with breakfast for example at 7:00, which you will have finished say at 7:30. Then the intake of calories is interrupted throughout the day and night until breakfast the following day at 7:00.

10 Myths About Fasting and Meal Frequency

Fasting has become increasingly common.

In fact, intermittent fasting, a dietary pattern that cycles between periods of fasting and eating, is often promoted as a miracle diet.

Yet, not everything you've heard about meal frequency and your health is true.

Here are 10 myths about fasting and meal frequency.

1. Skipping breakfast makes you fat

One ongoing myth is that breakfast is the most important meal of the day.

People commonly believe that skipping breakfast leads to excessive hunger, cravings, and weight gain.

One 16-week study in 283 adults with overweight and obesity observed no weight difference between those who ate breakfast and those who didn't .

Thus, breakfast doesn't largely affect your weight, although there may be some individual variability. Some studies even suggest that people who lose weight over the long term tend to eat breakfast .

What's more, children and teenagers who eat breakfast tend to perform better at school .

As such, it's important to pay attention to your specifc needs. Breakfast is beneficial for some people, while others can skip it without any negative consequences.

2. Eating frequently helps reduce hunger

Some people believe that periodic eating helps prevent cravings and excessive hunger.

Yet, the evidence is mixed.

Although some studies suggest that eating more frequent meals leads to reduced hunger, other studies have found no effect or even increased hunger levels.

One study that compared eating three or six high-protein meals per day found that eating three meals reduced hunger more effectively.

That said, responses may depend on the individual. If frequent eating reduces your cravings, it's probably a good idea. Still, there's no evidence that snacking or eating more often reduces hunger for everyone.

3. Eating frequently boosts your metabolism

Many people believe that eating more meals increases your metabolic rate, causing your body to burn more calories overall.

Your body indeed expends some calories digesting meals. This is termed the thermic effect of food TEF.

On average, TEF uses around 10% of your total calorie intake.

However, what matters is the total number of calories you consume — not how many meals you eat.

Eating six 500-calorie meals has the same effect as eating three 1,000-calorie meals. Given an average TEF of 10%, you'll burn 300 calories in both cases.

Numerous studies demonstrate that increasing or decreasing meal frequency does not affect total calories burned

4. Your brain needs a regular supply of dietary glucose

Some people claim that if you don't eat carbs every few hours, your brain will stop functioning.

This is based on the belief that your brain can only use glucose for fuel.

However, your body can easily produce the glucose it needs via a process called gluconeogenesis .

Even during long-term fasting, starvation, or very very-low-carb diets, your body can produce ketone bodies from dietary fats .

Ketone bodies can feed parts of your brain, reducing its glucose requirement significantly.

However, some people report feeling fatigued or shaky when they don't eat for a while. If this applies to you, you should consider keeping snacks on hand or eating more frequently

5. Frequent meals can help you lose weight

Since eating more frequently doesn't boost your metabolism, it likewise doesn't have any effect on weight loss .

Indeed, a study in 16 adults with obesity compared the effects of eating 3 and 6 meals per day and found no difference in weight, fat loss, or appetite .

Some people claim that eating often makes it harder for them to adhere to a healthy diet. However, if you find that eating more often makes it easier for you to eat fewer calories and less junk food, feel free to stick with it.

6. Fasting puts your body in starvation mode

One common argument against intermittent fasting is that it puts your body into starvation mode, thus shutting down your metabolism and preventing you from burning fat.

While it's true that long-term weight loss can reduce the number of calories you burn over time, this happens no matter what weight loss method you use .

There's no evidence that intermittent fasting causes a greater reduction in calories burned than other weight loss strategies.

In fact, short-term fasts may increase your metabolic rate.

This is due to a drastic increase in blood levels of norepinephrine, which stimulates your metabolism and instructs your fat cells to break down body fat.

Studies reveal that fasting for up to 48 hours can boost metabolism by 3.6–14%. However, if you fast much longer, the effects can reverse, decreasing your metabolism.

One study showed that fasting every other day for 22 days did not lead to a reduction in metabolic rate but a 4% loss of fat mass, on average.

7. Your body can only use a certain amount of protein per meal

Some people claim that you can only digest 30 grams of protein per meal and that you should eat every 2-3 hours to maximize muscle gain.

However, this is not supported by science.

Studies show that eating your protein in more frequent doses does not affect muscle mass.

The most important factor for most people is the total amount of protein consumed — not the number of meals it's spread over.

8. Intermittent fasting makes you lose muscle

Some people believe that when you fast, your body starts burning muscle for fuel.

Although this happens with dieting in general, no evidence suggests that it occurs more with intermittent fasting than other methods.

On the other hand, studies indicate that intermittent fasting is better for maintaining muscle mass.

In one review, intermittent fasting caused a similar amount of weight loss as continuous calorie restriction — but with much less reduction in muscle mass .

Another study showed a modest increase in muscle mass for people who consumed all their calories during one huge meal in the evening.

Notably, intermittent fasting is popular among many bodybuilders, who find that it helps maintain muscle alongside a low body fat percentage.

9. Intermittent fasting is bad for your health

While you may have heard rumors that intermittent fasting harms your health, studies reveal that it has several impressive health benefits .

For example, it changes your gene expression related to longevity and immunity and has been shown to prolong lifespan in animals.

It also has major benefits for metabolic health, such as improved insulin sensitivity and reduced oxidative stress, inflammation, and heart disease risk.

It may also boost brain health by elevating levels of brain-derived neurotrophic factor (BDNF), a hormone that may protect against depression and various other mental conditions

10. Intermittent fasting makes you overeat

Some individuals claim that intermittent fasting causes you to overeat during the eating periods.

While it's true that you may compensate for calories lost during a fast by automatically eating a little more afterward, this compensation isn't complete.

One study showed that people who fasted for 24 hours only ended up eating about 500 extra calories the next day — far fewer than the 2,400 calories they'd missed during the fat.

Because it reduces overall food intake and insulin levels while boosting metabolism, norepinephrine levels, and human growth hormone (HGH) levels, intermittent fasting makes you lose fat — not gain it.

According to one review, fasting for 3–24 weeks caused average weight and belly fat losses of 3–8% and 4–7%, respectively.

As such, intermittent fasting may be one of the most powerful tools to lose weight

What you can drink during intermittent fasting

You can drink it at will, indeed it is advisable. Also because good hydration accelerates the metabolism and reduces the sense of hunger. But not all drinks are good for this type of fasting.

The allowed drinks are (without sugar or sweeteners):

Water (possibly in a glass bottle or filtered with an active carbon filter)

Herbal tea (with water not from the tap)

Coffee

You

However, herbal teas, coffee and tea should not be sweetened with sweeteners containing sugar. If you can't do without it you can use some stevia to sweeten without calories and naturally.

The 6 Best Teas to Lose Weight and Belly Fat

Tea is a beverage enjoyed around the world.

You can make it by pouring hot water onto tea leaves and allowing them to steep for several minutes so their flavor infuses into the water.

This aromatic beverage is most commonly made from the leaves of Camellia sinensis, a type of evergreen shrub native to Asia.

Drinking tea has been associated with many health benefits, including protecting cells from damage and reducing the risk of heart disease

Some studies have even found that tea may enhance weight loss and help fight belly fat. Certain types have been found to be more effective than others at achieving this.

Below are six of the best teas for increasing weight loss and decreasing body fat.

1. Green Tea

Green tea is one of the most well-known types of tea, and is linked with many health benefits.

It's also one of the most effective teas for weight loss. There is substantial evidence linking green tea to decreases in both weight and body fat.

In one 2008 study, 60 obese people followed a standardized diet for 12 weeks while regularly drinking either green tea or a placebo.

Over the course of the study, those who drank green tea lost 7.3 pounds (3.3 kg) more weight than the placebo group .

Another study found that people who consumed green tea extract for 12 weeks experienced significant decreases in body weight, body fat and waist circumference, compared to a control group .

This may be because green tea extract is especially high in catechins, naturally occurring antioxidants that may boost your metabolism and increase fat burning.

This same effect also applies to matcha, a highly concentrated type of powdered green tea that contains the same beneficial ingredients as regular green tea.

2. Puerh Tea

Also known as pu'er or pu-erh tea, puerh tea is a type of Chinese black tea that has been fermented.

It is often enjoyed after a meal, and has an earthy aroma that tends to develop the longer it's stored.

Some animal studies have shown that puerh tea may lower blood sugar and blood triglycerides. And studies in animals and humans have shown that puerh tea may be able to help enhance weight loss.

In one study, 70 men were given either a capsule of puerh tea extract or a placebo. After three months, those taking the puerh tea capsule lost approximately 2.2 pounds (1 kg) more than the placebo group.

Another study in rats had similar findings, showing that puerh tea extract had an anti-obesity effect and helped suppress weight gain .

Current research is limited to puerh tea extract, so more research is needed to see if the same effects apply to drinking it as a tea.

3. Black Tea

Black tea is a type of tea that has undergone more oxidation than other types, such as green, white or oolong teas.

Oxidation is a chemical reaction that happens when the tea leaves are exposed to the air, resulting in browning that causes the characteristic dark color of black tea.

There are many different types and blends of black tea available, including popular varieties like Earl Grey and English breakfast.

Several studies have found that black tea could be effective when it comes to weight control.

One study of 111 people found that drinking three cups of black tea each day for three months significantly increased weight loss and reduced waist circumference, compared to drinking a caffeine-matched control beverage.

Some theorize that black tea's potential weight loss effects may be because it's high in flavones, a type of plant pigment with antioxidant properties.

A study followed 4,280 adults over 14 years. It found that those with a higher flavone intake from foods and beverages like black tea had a lower body mass index (BMI) than those with a lower flavone intake.

However, this study looks only at the association between BMI and flavone intake. Further research is needed to account for other factors that may be involved.

4. Oolong Tea

Oolong tea is a traditional Chinese tea that has been partially oxidized, putting it somewhere between green tea and black tea in terms of oxidation and color.

It is often described as having a fruity, fragrant aroma and a unique flavor, though these can vary significantly depending on the level of oxidation.

Several studies have shown that oolong tea could help enhance weight loss by improving fat burning and speeding up metabolism.

In one study, 102 overweight or obese people drank oolong tea every day for six weeks, which may have helped reduce both their body weight and body fat. The researchers proposed the tea did this by improving the metabolism of fat in the body .

Another small study gave men either water or tea for a three-day period, measuring their metabolic rates. Compared to water, oolong tea increased energy expenditure by 2.9%, the equivalent of burning an additional 281 calories per day, on average .

While more studies on the effects of oolong tea are needed, these findings show that oolong could be potentially beneficial for weight loss.

5. White Tea

White tea stands out among other types of tea because it is minimally processed and harvested while the tea plant is still young.

White tea has a distinct flavor very different from other types of tea. It tastes subtle, delicate and slightly sweet.

The benefits of white tea are well-studied, and range from improving oral health to killing cancer cells in some test-tube studies.

Though further research is needed, white tea could also help when it comes to losing weight and body fat.

Studies show that white tea and green tea have comparable amounts of catechins, which may help enhance weight loss .

Furthermore, one test-tube study showed that white tea extract increased the breakdown of fat cells while preventing the formation of new ones .

However, keep in mind that this was a test-tube study, so it's unclear how the effects of white tea may apply to humans.

Additional studies are needed to confirm the potential beneficial effects of white tea when it comes to fat loss.

6. Herbal Tea

Herbal teas involve the infusion of herbs, spices and fruits in hot water.

They differ from traditional teas because they do not typically contain caffeine, and are not made from the leaves of Camellia sinensis.

Popular herbal tea varieties include rooibos tea, ginger tea, rosehip tea and hibiscus tea.

Although the ingredients and formulations of herbal teas can vary significantly, some studies have found that herbal teas may help with weight reduction and fat loss.

In one animal study, researchers gave obese rats an herbal tea, and found that it reduced body weight and helped normalize hormone levels.

Rooibos tea is a type of herbal tea that may be especially effective when it comes to fat burning.

One test-tube study showed that rooibos tea increased fat metabolism and helped block the formation of fat cells.

However, further studies in humans are needed to look into the effects of herbal teas like rooibos on weight loss

Though many people drink tea solely for its soothing quality and delicious taste, each cup may also pack many health benefits.

Replacing high-calorie beverages like juice or soda with tea could help reduce overall calorie intake and lead to weight loss.

Some animal and test-tube studies have also shown that certain types of tea may help increase weight loss while blocking fat cell formation. However, studies in humans are needed to investigate this further.

Additionally, many types of tea are especially high in beneficial compounds like flavones and catechins, which could aid in weight loss as well.

Coupled with a healthy diet and regular exercise, a cup or two of tea each day could help you boost weight loss and prevent harmful belly fat

How many times you have to do intermittent fasting

Now that you understand how to implement an intermittent fasting schedule, it raises a question: How often should you fast?

The answer varies from individual to individual. Most individuals implement the above schedules every week or every other week. If you're new to fasting, start with a moderate schedule, trying it every other week or every three weeks. If your body adapts well, aim for a regular, weekly schedule.

There's no wrong answer here. Pay close attention to how your body responds to your fasting schedule, and adjust as needed. Keep in mind that life changes can happen. You may need to tweak your schedule to allow for social gatherings, vacations and physical activity or competition.

In general, once or twice a week is an optimal frequency to perform intermittent fasting.

What not to eat during intermittent fasting

Any source of calories should be avoided during the period of intermittent fasting. So also all the oils and obviously sugars.

Any solid food should be avoided, including fruits, seeds and vegetables. Even shredded versions, extracts and juices are NOT used during the period of intermittent fasting.

Who should not do intermittent fasting

If you suffer or have suffered from eating disorders, it is not recommended to face any type of calorie restriction.

It is not appropriate for children to follow an intermittent fast.

Women in general should address it in the less aggressive version by 16 hours no more than 1-2 times a week. In fact, some women may be affected by hormonal changes (increased testosterone) which could lead to amenorrhea.

If the woman suffers from infertility she should avoid intermittent fasting.

In any case of pre-existing conditions it is necessary to discuss with your doctor to see if in the specific case it is advantageous to deal with the practice of intermittent fasting.

Who can deal with intermittent fasting

In general, boys are the ones who only benefit from intermittent fasting.

All people (except children) are healthy, especially if overweight can benefit enormously from intermittent fasting.

As indicated in the initial part of the article, the human being in the course of its evolution has always had to confront the lack of food. Eating less and less often is one of the most natural and healthy things there is.

The problem today is rather in the sense of excess. How many diseases are caused by unhealthy foods consumed in excess!

Intermittent fasting is the (simple) turn we need

... It is appropriate to correct this trend as soon as possible by turning to the healthy habit of intermittently fasting.

There is a way of saying oriental wisdom that suggests ...

"No matter how far you've gotten away from the right path ... turn!"

The important thing is to correct yourself and do it immediately.

The more you continue in the same (wrong) direction under the influence of inertia, the more you will drift away: turning, now!

Conclusions

Are you lazy but want to do something more to regain health and fitness?

Intermittent fasting has all the characteristics to unleash a great therapeutic, protective and slimming power.

There is nothing healthier, simpler and cheaper than to stop eating for 16-24 hours 1-2 times a week. You can also count the 7-8 hours of sleep in the total number of intermittent fasting hours (so in the easiest version it is like fasting for only 8 hours!).

On the practical side, fasting intermittently also facilitates life. In fact, skipping a couple of meals every now and then eliminates the need to prepare them and you recover some time to devote to something else.

Motivation: Intermittet fasting success stories
Intermittent Fasting Success Stories

1. lucy's Story

After one year of 4:3 intermittent fasting, I've lost 39.8kg (6 stone 3.8lb). My body mass index (BMI) has reduced by 12.28, down to 36.79 from 49.07. I have had to throw many of my old clothes out because they have become loose and comical.

During the second half of my fasting (the latter six months of the twelve), I experienced long plateau periods, meaning little weight loss was apparent due to my metabolism slowing and my body burning fewer calories, strangely, these plateaus seem to only occur when approaching a weight-loss milestone

(130kgs, 120kgs), and were usually followed by an abrupt and substantial loss of weight. Whilst I am aware that plateau is quite common around the six to nine-month mark of dieting, I am hoping to get past it and speed up my weight loss process.

I find it is easy to do after a year. On most fasting days, I often eat nothing at all, and sometimes continue the fasting until my afternoon meal the next day if I am not overly hungry.

All in all, I feel fantastic, although I still carry a lot of body weight, I feel much lighter on my feet and more energetic than I was before. I also feel as though my strength and endurance have improved.

2. Tabatha's Story

I have had to throw all of my old clothes out and purchase an entirely new wardrobe since fasting. I have just turned 65, my weight is now 127lbs, my body-fat ratio is 27.3%, I have a BMI of 20.2%, and a 29-inch waistline. I am feeling very good and am planning on continuing my dietary plan for a few years or more, to ensure I remain healthy and enjoy the years I have left to the fullest.Here's how I achieved it:

I use the 5:2 method, whereby I only had to count calories on two days out of seven in a week.During the early stages of the regime I would nibble on snacks the evening before fast days to load up on calories, and the next day whilst fasting I would be thinking about food non-stop. However, this didn't last that long, and it wasn't long before I stopped snacking even on non-fasting days.

I found that distributing my calorie intake between the times of 12 pm and 7 pm, and skipping breakfast everyday (as I had always struggled to consume and enjoy breakfast consistently) worked wonders for me.

Once I hit my target weight in March, I decided to change to a 6:1 plan to see how my body would react. What I found was that even when I didn't fast at all throughout the week by adhering to the 7-hour window (between 12 pm and 7 pm), I was still steadily losing weight. After reading some intermittent fasting success stories, I found that this seven-hour window had been useful for others, too.

After going on holiday, I put on a few pounds, but once I had returned home and re-established my seven hour eating window, I lost the extra holiday weight within two weeks.

3. Jina's Story

After deciding that it was time to change my eating habits and attain what is considered a healthy weight for my age, I decided to try 5:2 intermittent fasting. I began fasting on the 1st of July 2013, and my body weight was 170lbs (12st 2lbs), as of today (September 24th, 2013), my body weight has dropped to 145lbs (10st 5lbs).

I generally fast on Mondays, Thursdays, or Fridays, depending on impending commitments. I fast from evening meal to evening meal, for 24 hour periods. At one point I attempted to fast for a 36-hour period, but this caused me to have trouble sleeping and left my stomach feeling extremely empty. For this reason, I continued to consume a small, nutritious meal in the evening on fast days.

I began diet by eating complex carbohydrates (whole meal bread, spaghetti, and brown rice), but have swapped these starchy foods for courgette "spaghetti" and cauliflower "rice", which are delicious alternatives. I have abstained from eating all white carbohydrates, and I log everything I eat into an app on my smart phone which records the calorie content. This provides me with helpful statistics and ensures I adhere to my weight loss goals.

Since fasting I have gone from a size 16 to a size 10, and I am feeling very positive about my appearance. I have read many intermittent fasting success stories to ascertain that I am not alone in my success. I will continue to maintain my fasting plan and work toward my target weight of 139lbs (9st 13lbs).

4. Maria's Story

After putting a few stone on during menopause, I decided to try intermittent fasting to lose my post-menopausal weight. Starting in September/October time in 2012, I first implemented the 5:2 diet plan but soon began a 16/8 method, wherein I would have 16 hour fast periods and 8 hour eating windows every day. I get great displeasure from counting calories so I found this method best suited for more – simply skip breakfast and don't nibble in the evenings, how hard could it be? Since fasting I have gone from 140lbs (10st) to around 112/117lbs (8st to 8st 4lbs).

At first I would eat whatever I wanted during the 8 hour eating period of each day, with little to no concern of healthy/nutritious meals. Before long, I began to implement healthier meals and really noticed the benefits from doing so.

At first, weight loss was slow, which can be disheartening, but I persevered and eventually lost the weight I wanted to. I feel brilliant, full of energy and life, and my friends and family say I look better than I have for many years. Intermittent fasting truly has changed my life for the better. I would definitely recommend this method of eating, and this way of life to anyone.

AUTOPHAGY GUIDE Introduction

Autophagy is a natural process that occurs in our bodies continuously from birth. Our bodies use this process to recycle cells and their components. But even though autophagy is a cleanup process that happens all the time, now we have the knowledge to harness its power and tap its benefits when we want to. In the following article, we explain what autophagy is, and how to induce it when you want to experience its benefits.

What is autophagy?

You might have heard of autophagy before. You might even know people who say that this process helped them lose weight. But how can autophagy help someone lose weight since it's basically a natural cleaning process? Let's find out.

The Autophagy Definition
If you pick up a biology manual or look up autophagy in search engines – do people

still use manuals these days? -, you might get a response similar to the one below:

Autophagy is the natural process by which cellular material is degraded by lysosomes or vacuoles. This mechanism is induced by specific pathways such as chaperone-mediated autophagy, macroautophagy, and microautophagy. Now, this definition is very technical, but it's also very difficult to understand. Sure, we might understand some of the words, but what do they actually mean? Let's break it down.

Autophagy is a process in which cells eat themselves (in Greek, the term literally means self-eating). All cells degrade at certain rates. For example, a red blood cell lives on average 115 days. The cells on the top layer of our skin usually live 14 – 30 days, whereas neurons can live for years.

But the human body is extremely efficient, and it doesn't want to lose all the components of the dead cells, or the damaged components of living cells only to create them again from scratch for new cells that serve the same purpose.

This is where the lysosomes come in. These organelles break down the cells and they recycle all the useful components like protein while eliminating intracellular pathogens such as bacteria or viruses. They dispose of the cells' dysfunctional parts. We'll talk more about why this important below.

Selective Types of Autophagy:

The focus of this special issue of the International Journal of Cell Biology is to underscore the recent developments in the field of macroautophagy and how this degradative pathway intersects with cellular metabolism, complex physiological functions, and human diseases. During the last decade, autophagy has become an expanding field in biomedical life sciences due to its involvement with numerous intracellular processes. Autophagy also plays a role in pathology, and it has the therapeutic potential to be the target for the treatment of specific human diseases. Early studies suggested that autophagy was a nonselective process in which cytoplasmic structures were randomly sequestered into autophagosomes before being delivered to the mammalian lysosome or the plant and yeast vacuole for degradation. Now there is growing evidence that unwanted cellular structures can be selectively recognized and exclusively eliminated within cells (F. Reggiori et al., "Selective types of autophagy"). This is achieved through the action of specific autophagy receptors, as reviewed by C. Behrends and S. Fulda in "Receptor proteins in selective autophagy") and studied by K. Marchbank et al. "MAP1B interaction with the FW domain of the autophagic receptor Nbr1 facilitates its association to the microtubule network". Thus excess or damaged organelles including mitochondria (A. May et al., "The many faces of mitochondrial autophagy: making sense of contrasting observations in recent research"; Y. Hirota et al., "The physiological role of mitophagy: new insights into phosphorylation events"), peroxisomes (A. Till et al., "Pexophagy: the selective degradation of peroxisomes"), lipid droplets (R. Singh and A. Cuervo, "Lipophagy: connecting autophagy and lipid metabolism"), endoplasmic reticulum and ribosomes (E.

Cebollero et al., "Reticulophagy and ribophagy: regulated degradation of protein production factories") can be specifically sequestered by autophagosomes and targeted to the lysosome for degradation.

Importantly, there is growing evidence that selective autophagy subtypes also have a wide range of physiological functions. In yeast, the cytosol-to-vacuole (Cvt) pathway transports hydrolases into the vacuole, which is reviewed by M. Umekawa and D. Klionsky in "The cytoplasm-to-vacuole targeting pathway: a historical perspective". In eukaryotes, autophagy plays a central role in both innate and acquired immunity. Further sequestration and elimination of invading pathogens such as Salmonella and Staphylococcus aureus have been exploited to study autophagosome biogenesis (T. Noda et al., "Three-axis model for Atg recruitment in autophagy against Salmonella"; M. Mauthe et al., "WIPI-1 positive autophagosome-like vesicles entrap pathogenic Staphylococcus aureus for lysosomal degradation"). In pancreas cells, autophagy has recently been shown to specifically turn over secretory granules, as described by M. Vaccaro in "Zymophagy: selective autophagy of secretory granules". Dysregulation of autophagic function has been implicated in a growing list of disease processes and has underscored the selective or substrate-specific versions of the pathway. Examples in this special issue include the clearance of aggregates associated with neurological diseases, as reviewed by T. Lamark and T. Johansen in "Aggrephagy: selective disposal of protein aggregates by macroautophagy" and by I. Nezis in "Selective autophagy in Drosophila". In terms of cancer biology, autophagy has been viewed as having dual roles in both tumor suppression and progression. K. Hughson et al. in "Implications of therapy-induced selective autophagy on tumor metabolism and survival" review how activation of autophagy selective forms can be used as a potential therapeutic approach for the treatment of specific cancers. Adding to the complexity of autophagic function and regulation, the article by K. Juenemann and E. Reits "Alternative macroautophagic pathways" explores alternative macroautophagic pathways that are independent of key core autophagy components such as Beclin-1 or Atg5. We expect future research on the mechanism and regulation of selective autophagy, and the physiological importance of this pathway in human disease will be very exciting and expand on the findings highlighted in this issue of IJC

The History of Autophagy

In 1963, Christian de Duve, a Belgian scientist was studying the effects of insulin on the liver when he stumbled upon a process nobody has documented before. He noticed that some cells cannibalized parts of their own structure in a presumed cleanup process. Thanks to de Duve's findings, the connection autophagy – lysosome was made.

Even though the Belgian scientist's discovery happened in the '60s and had lead to de Duve's Nobel Prize in 1974, it wasn't until the '80s that researchers really understood its importance.

The breakthrough came in 1983 when Japanese biologist Yoshinori Ohsumi discovered that specific genes regulate autophagy. He discovered that autophagy doesn't happen without the help of these genes, which means that cells can't repair themselves and the body doesn't recycle as many components when the cell dies. This discovery led to Ohsumi's Nobel Prize in 2016 and an important Breakthrough Prize in Life Sciences in 2017.

The Possible Benefits of Autophagy

You might be wondering what makes autophagy so important. Well, according to the latest studies – and there have been thousands of articles published on autophagy until now – stimulating this process might produce a lot of benefits. Here is a list of the most important ones.

It May Extend Aging

Autophagy is important because it allows the body to reuse some of the cell's components, but it's also one of the ways the cell can actually repair itself. As cells age, they lose some of their functions. This is a natural process, one that's directly correlated to the cells' functional components. In truth, aging could be defined as the accumulation of different forms of molecular damage.

A cell accumulates its damaged components until a lysosome disposes of them. At the same time, the likelihood of developing chronic diseases such as diabetes or even cancer increases concomitantly with the accumulated damage.

By triggering the autophagy, the lysosome is removing the dysfunctional components, reducing their harmful potential. Since the cleanup process removes the damaged parts of the cell, it actually manages to prevent the development of diseases. And it gets better. Since aging could be defined as

the sum of the cells' molecular damage,
removing the damaged cells' components
might actually delay the aging process
itself.

Protects Against Psychiatric Disorders

Neurodegeneration is the leading cause of
mental illness. And unfortunately, brain
diseases are often difficult to treat.
Neurons might be considered the most
important cells in the body, but they still
suffer damage every day. Sometimes,
neural degradation is caused by the
accumulation of proteins, while other
times the neurons might be affected by a
virus or bacteria. When a sufficient
number of neurons are damaged, they

start behaving erratically, leading to clinical manifestations of various psychiatric disorders.

However, recent studies suggest that autophagy might be an efficient way of preventing the onset of psychiatric diseases. Autophagy preserves the balance between the degradation of existing neurons, the recycling of their useful components, and the creation of new ones.

Those who suffer from schizophrenia show a deficiency in their autophagy pathways. Simply put, for those who suffer from schizophrenia, the autophagy process is not triggered at the right time. This creates an imbalance between the death of existing neurons and the creation of new ones, which leads to the disease's onset.

Prevents Neurodegenerative Disorders

You might have noticed that we talked about neural degradation caused by the accumulation of proteins. Well, this determines Alzheimer's, Parkinson's, and Huntington's diseases. The neurons of those who suffer from these diseases are assaulted by abnormal proteins called prions.

The accumulation of protein in the brain leads to profound changes in thinking and behavior and ultimately leads to the development of neurodegenerative diseases.

Autophagy increases the clearance of abnormal protein, as well as that of infectious and toxic agents. By triggering the autophagy process, researchers believe we might actually prevent the accumulation of both infectious and inflammatory agents that determine neurodegenerative diseases.

It Helps Fight Infectious Diseases

Autophagy can prevent the development of infectious diseases, and it can help fight the disease if you already contacted it. And the great thing is, this natural cleanup process is actually better at fighting infection than you would think.

You certainly heard of tuberculosis. Tuberculosis (or TB) is a disease that caused 1.3 million deaths worldwide in 2016 alone. You definitely know all about HIV, as well. These diseases are responsible for millions of deaths worldwide, and both of them can be prevented by autophagy.

When the lysosome triggers the autophagy mechanism, it targets the foreign and damaged components it finds in the cell for removal. The lysosome is so apt at removing the harmful components, it can degrade both the HIV virus and the TB bacteria so that they can't multiply and spread inside the body.

Regulates Inflammation

Autophagy helps regulate the body's inflammatory response. In fact, this is one of the mechanisms responsible for presenting the harmful particle to the immune cells which leads to the onset of the immune response.

And autophagy can also reduce the inflammatory response. All the foreign particles that enter the body are capable of launching an immune response. Even a damaged cell component can trigger an immune response if it's not cleared in a timely manner. By constantly removing these particles, the cleaning process helps regulate the inflammatory response.

Improves Muscle Performance

If you didn't spend the last two decades or so in a cave, you might have heard that exercise is good for your health. When we train our muscles, the exercises actually cause a trauma to the skeletal muscle fibers. The trauma determines an intervention of the immune system that triggers an inflammatory response. The inflammation contains and repairs the damage, and helps clean up the waste products in the area.

And as you probably guessed by now, the autophagy mechanism helps clean up the waste products as well. This mechanism is actually the one responsible for a low to moderate immune response. If the autophagy wouldn't step in to clean up the waste products, the immune response would be greater and potentially dangerous.

But the autophagy process improves our muscle performance in more ways than one.

Even though they might not be useful, the damaged components of the cell still consume energy. By eliminating and recycling the damaged components, the autophagy helps the cell optimize its energy use and minimize its energy waste.

Can Help With Cancer Prevention

Chronic inflammation is one of the leading factors in cancer development. When a harmful particle abuses a cell, the body launches an inflammatory response.

Sometimes, the inflammatory response cannot subdue the harmful agent in a timely manner. This leads to a chronic inflammation. Since the harmful agent is still present in the body, it can still produce toxins that can accumulate and lead to cancer.

Autophagy is helpful because it can help remove the harmful agent. Sometimes, even though it can't remove the agent, the cleanup process will prevent the toxin accumulation, lowering the stress the body faces. This allows it to suppress the cancer initiation.

Enhances Metabolic Efficiency

Autophagy eliminates all the cells' damaged components, preventing them from using energy needlessly. This will optimize the cells' energy use, which will make them stronger and more resilient. And a good thing about this cleanup process is that it's highly adaptable. If the body is facing a stressful situation, the autophagy mechanism will regulate the energy use by eliminating the cells' components that are unnecessary.

How to Induce Autophagy

Now that we've listed the most important benefits of autophagy, let's take a look at how to stimulate this process.

Autophagy Fasting

Our bodies perceive fasting as stress. And that makes sense when you think about it. When you're fasting, you're hungry, moody, and your body will make efforts to optimize your energy distribution. And that's precisely what makes fasting a perfect trigger for autophagy. Now, before we proceed and explain how to use fasting to trigger autophagy, let's take a look at the different types of fasts you can choose from.

Long Fasts – These types of fasts require you to abstain from food for at least 24 hours.

Dry Fast – Despite its harshness, this is still a popular type of fast. The dry fast is extremely dangerous because you don't get to eat OR drink anything. Abstaining from drinking water is not advisable by any means. We do not recommend this fast. In fact, we recommend you avoid it, for your own sake.

Water Fast – Another popular type of fast, the water fast has been researched for its value in weight loss. This fast requires you to abstain from eating anything, but it allows and even recommends drinking water. Some people have adapted this fast, and they consume juices or protein shakes instead of water. While these methods might be effective for weight loss – even though multiple studies indicated that juicing is actually harmful to the body and is NOT indicated for weight loss – they are not true facts because you consume calories.

Long fasts promote weight loss and autophagy. A single 24-hour fast can reverse the loss of stem cell function, which will dramatically improve their regeneration capacities.

You might be wondering how long you have to fast to stimulate autophagy – well, most studies agree that a period of 24-hours would suffice. Some studies indicate that a fasting period of 16 hours would also stimulate the autophagy process, which suggests that time-restricted and intermittent fasting are viable options.

Even though some studies found that time-restricted and intermittent fasting are viable options to trigger autophagy, they are not as reliable as the long fasts. If you want to make sure you stimulate the process, abstain from eating for a period of 24 – 36 hours. Keep in mind that fasting is about avoiding calories. That doesn't mean you shouldn't drink water, tea, or coffee, as long as you don't add any sugar or other sweeteners to them.

Ketogenic Diet

Autophagy

One of the benefits of the ketogenic diet is that it limits your calorie consumption without limiting your food intake. This diet requires you to consume at least 75 percent of your calories from fat and refrain from consuming more than ten percent from carbohydrates. Your body prefers to use the glucose extracted from carbohydrates as fuel, but if it doesn't find any carbs easily available, it changes its metabolic pathways and uses ketones extracted from fat as fuel instead.

Now, this shift might seem important to those who want to lose weight, but where does autophagy fit into this scenario?

Well, this shift actually happens naturally when we fast. The human body is highly adaptable. When we fast, our bodies look for other energy sources besides glucose, and they start breaking down fat to overcome starvation. This process is called ketogenesis. When the body is in a ketogenic state, the autophagy process is stimulated to optimize the cells' energy consumption and improve the body's energy output.

The ketogenic diet triggers the same process to help us lose weight. But the great thing about this diet is that you don't have to starve yourself to trigger ketogenesis. This makes the ketogenic diet a viable option for those who are unable to fast.

Exercise

Physical exercise stimulates the autophagy process. Exercise stimulated autophagy in multiple tissues and organs, such as the liver, pancreas, muscle, and adipose tissue. Surprisingly, exercise-induced autophagy in the cerebral cortex.

Even though this aspect is not fully understood at the moment, it strengthens researchers' belief that regular exercise could prevent the onset of neurodegenerative diseases such as Alzheimer's or Parkinson's. In addition, it seems like the exercise-induced autophagy helped with the development of new neurons and it helped improve the cognitive function. The process also optimized the energy consumption of the liver and pancreatic cells.

BENEFICIAL EFFECTS OF EXERCISE ON NAFLD

Changes in lifestyle such as weight loss and dietary modification have long been established as the first step in the management of NAFLD. Weight loss seems to independently improve hepatic function in NAFLD, although improved profile of intrahepatic lipids requires at least 3%–5% weight loss through physical activity and calorie control. Exercise alters various biochemical activities not only in the muscle, but also in the liver and adipose tissue. The muscle-liver cross talk in energy and metabolic balance also is inferred from the observation that the patients with CLD manifest a higher incidence of sarcopenia, a loss of muscle mass. A recent study further suggests a strong association between sarcopenia and NAFLD in both nonobese and obese subjects. The importance of muscle-liver cross talk also is implicated in a transgenic animal study where genetic ablation of myostatin, a TGF-β superfamily member that regulates skeletal muscle mass, ameliorated high fat diet–induced elevation of liver weight (51). Considering multiple benefits on the metabolic syndrome by increasing physical activity, it has been proposed that the skeletal muscle could be a pharmacological target for treating metabolic disorders including NAFLD.

How exercise directly or indirectly diminishes intrahepatic lipids independently of diet modification, however, remains unclear. The simplest view could be mobilization of hepatic lipids to the muscle to fuel muscular energy deficit during physical activity. Exercise increases glucose uptake in the muscles and concomitantly signals the liver to enhance glucose production to support continued energy expenditure. The demand for increased gluconeogenesis further stimulates the degradation of intracellular lipids to provide mitochondrial substrates for β-oxidation. Besides enhancing free fatty acid oxidation in mitochondria, physical activity, particularly chronic aerobic exercise, also may reduce hepatic lipogenesis. In a high fat–fed mouse model, treadmill exercise substantially decreases the expression of sterol regulatory element-binding protein-1c, a transcription factor triggering triglyceride synthesis. Chronic consumption of high fat or high carbohydrate diet elevates levels of inflammatory cytokines such as tumor necrosis factor (TNF) α and interleukin-1β . We previously have shown that in the livers of old rats there was a significant increase in nuclear presence of nuclear factor κB and several other proteins, demonstrating an increased pro-inflammatory response. The age-associated increase in the upregulation of pro-inflammatory proteins was substantially attenuated in the livers of old animals exposed to long-term voluntary exercise by wheel running. Although physical exercise may attenuate hepatic inflammation by reducing pro-inflammatory cytokines, the mechanisms of anti-inflammatory benefits by exercise remain to be elucidated.

Using a mouse treadmill model, He et al.recently showed that physical activity stimulates autophagy in a wide range of tissues, including the skeletal muscle, heart, liver, pancreas, and adipose tissue. The exercise-mediated autophagy induction likely is to occur at the initiation step of autophagy through the dissociation of BECN1 from BCL2. Mice lacking three conserved phosphorylation sites of Thr69, Ser70, and Ser97 in the nonstructured loop of BCL2 failed to induce autophagy after exercise. Furthermore, these genetically modified animals were unable to run on a treadmill as long as their wild-type counterparts, implying that BECN1-dependent autophagy may be uniquely launched by exercise. Intriguingly, analysis of p62 and LC3-II/LC3-I, markers of autophagy induction, revealed that exercise also markedly increases autophagy in extramuscular tissues such as the liver and pancreas, although no apparent morphological or structural alterations were observed in hepatocytes and pancreatic β-cells from the mice expressing nonphosphoryltable BCL2. In particular, long-term exercise ameliorated high fat diet–induced glucose intolerance in wild-type mice but not in BCL2 mutant mice, substantiating the importance of autophagy in exercise-mediated cytoprotection against metabolic disorder.

Taken together, this study demonstrates that exercise is a natural stimulus of autophagy that can confer metabolic protection.

How the muscle transduces an autophagy initiation signal to the liver is currently unknown. The skeletal muscle is an endocrine organ secreting a plethora of cytokines, chemokines, growth factors, hormones, and vasoactive factors, collectively termed myokines. Autophagy induction after physical training might involve these myokines. Myonectin or C1q/TNF-related protein 5 (CTRP5) is a nutrient-responsive myokine that enhances glucose uptake and stimulates fatty acid oxidation. This myokine often is released in response to feeding and insulin. Interestingly, exogenous administration of recombinant CTRP5 to the liver and cultured hepatocytes has been shown to prevent autophagy via activating mTOR pathway. Using a high fat diet rodent model, Lei et al. demonstrated that CTRP5-null animals exhibit reduced hepatic steatosis and improved insulin action, implying a negative correlation between CTRP5 and NAFLD onset. Intriguingly, aerorobic exercise has been reported to diminish levels of CTRP5 in humans. Although future studies are warranted to determine how this muscle-derived cytokine is delivered to and triggers autophagic signals in the liver, these studies suggest that hepatic autophagy could be modulated by the changes in CTRP5 levels after physical activity

Other myokines also might mediate autophagy stimulation in the liver. Irisin, an active form of the fibronectin type III domain containing 5 protein, is a newly identified exercise-induced myokine. Irisin activates AMPK signaling in hepatocytes and reduces intracellular triglyceride accumulation. Because AMPK is an essential player in autophagy initiation, irisin derived from the muscle might be an important signaling molecule that translocates to the liver and stimulates hepatic signaling of autophagy (Figure). However, it is important to note that despite numerous studies, large controversy still exists as to how much irisin increases after exercise in humans. Tandem mass spectrometric analysis of 10 individuals found that high intensity aerobic exercise increases the level of circulating irisin by 19%. Although statistically significant, this elevation is rather small. Future studies are required with larger populations of subjects to investigate how various exercise conditions affect irisin production in humans and how the liver interacts with this myokine released from the muscle.

Reduced calorie intake without malnutrition or calorie restriction (CR) has long been shown to effectively expand lifespan in various species including primates. One potential mechanism of

CR-mediated benefit may be its induction of autophagy. Several studies have demonstrated that chronic or long-term CR facilitates protein turnover by activating multiple regulatory pathways of autophagy. For instance, CR acts on the upstream events of autophagy initiation by suppressing mTORC1 and stimulating AMPK, which in turn leads to ULK1 activation. Furthermore, CR enhances sirtuin 1 activity, an enzyme that induces autophagy through deacetylating multiple cellular targets. Although autophagy evidently is launched by either CR or exercise, ongoing controversies exist as to whether the combination of dietary intervention with exercise could provide greater benefits than CR or exercise alone

Although resistance exercise increases the strength and cross-sectional area of muscle fibers, endurance exercise, also known as aerobic exercise, augments the mitochondrial function and content of the muscle. Although either type of exercise profoundly influences cellular protein turnover, accumulating evidence indicates differential effects on protein homeostasis between resistance and endurance exercise. Within 24 h after acute endurance exercise, messenger RNA of key autophagy factors, including LC3, ATG4B, ATG12, BNIP3, and cathepsin L, is upregulated. A study with a mouse model of 40-min exercise duration showed that moderate-to-low intensity exercise rapidly promotes the phosphorylation of the residues of Ser317 and 555 of ULK1, while preventing mTORC1-dependent ULK1 phosphorylation, events indicative of autophagy initiation. It is, however, noteworthy that the increase in autophagy in response to a common endurance exercise is not always observed in other studies wherein animals are exposed to 50 to 90 min of tread mill exercise. This could imply that exercise duration may be an important factor contributing to autophagy induction in the muscle. Another important factor in endurance exercise–mediated autophagy induction is a feeding status before exercise. When autophagy onset during endurance exercise is compared between fast and fed state, stimulation of autophagy becomes more robust in the fasted state, as evidenced by a higher increase in LC3, BNIP3, and Parkin

In contrast with endurance exercise, a decrease in autophagy has been reported after resistance exercise. In humans, although resistance exercise reduces the lipidation of LC3-I, an integral event for autophagy induction, E3-ligase activity in the ubiquitin-proteasome pathway seems to be upregulated after this exercise regimen. Increased expression of class III PI3K has been reported after resistance exercise. However, because this kinase also is involved in multiple pathways other than autophagy, these studies do not necessarily reflect autophagy involvement in response to resistance exercise. Although current literatures favor nonessential roles of autophagy in strength and resistance exercise, future studies are needed to clarify better how autophagy is associated with this exercise regimen. It also is important to understand potential impacts of a combination of resistance and endurance exercise on muscle autophagy

EFFECTS OF MUSCLE AUTOPHAGY ON THE LIVER

Growing evidence supports the presence of a remote communication between individual organs. The skeletal muscles are a major provider of gluconeogenic and ketogenic amino acids during prolonged starvation in mammals. Because the liver is a primary tissue controlling both gluconeogenesis and ketogenesis and starvation is a powerful autophagy inducer in the liver and muscle as well, it is plausible to speculate that muscle autophagy could impact the liver directly or vice versa. Although defective autophagy in the muscle causes accumulation of intramyocellular triglycerides and enhanced autophagy facilitates removal of lipids from muscle cells, Takagi et al. recently demonstrated in tissue-specific ATG5 knockout mice that the mice lacking ATG5 in both the liver and muscle indeed exhibited the improvement of metabolic profile, compared with liver-specific knockout counterparts, suggesting that autophagy in the skeletal muscle metabolically may be distinct from that in the liver. In an independent study, skeletal muscle–specific ATG7 knockout mice also showed lower lipid accumulation and higher expression of β-oxidation–related genes, compared with control mice . Furthermore, when fed with high fat diet, these transgenic animals displayed lower expression of lipogenic genes in the liver and were protected from diet-induced obesity and insulin resistance. Because high fat diet markedly causes accumulation of lipid droplets in the autophagy-deficient livers, it is likely that metabolic outcomes after the onset of autophagy or lipophagy in the muscle may be different from those in the liver

Sleep

Even though most of us give up sleep to watch their favorite series, work more, or spend time with friends, our bodies function best when we respect their natural clocks or circadian rhythms. Our biological clock controls our sleep cycles, but it seems it controls the autophagy process as well.

Respecting our circadian rhythm is very important because it actually controls our metabolism. Our bodies order the production and release of hormones while we sleep. The lack of sleep is considered a stressful activity, and it has adverse effects on our health and wellbeing.

And sleep is also necessary to induce autophagy. The lack of sleep disturbs the autophagy process, and it slows it down considerably.

Autophagy boosting foods

Eating certain foods can stimulate the autophagy process. Here is a list of the most efficient foods you can eat to induce this cleaning process.

Coffee

Several studies suggested that coffee consumption could inhibit several metabolic diseases. Now, it seems that coffee is so effective at reducing the incidence of metabolic diseases because it increases the autophagy process throughout the body.

And the best part is, you don't have to abuse caffeine to benefit from these effects. Scientists have noticed an increased autophagy in the heart, liver, and muscle cells after the consumption of a single coffee cup.

Ginger

Ginger consumption can induce autophagy. The active component of ginger, called 6-shogaol, can induce an autophagy process that's so powerful it can actually help destroy a type of lung cancer cells.

Green Tea

Some of the active ingredients found in green tea can stimulate the autophagy process in the liver cells. EGCG, a polyphenol commonly found in green and white tea can induce the autophagy in the liver. This process is helpful against inflammation, cancer, and liver damage.

Coconut Oil

Coconut oil contains a lot of ketones, the same components the body produces naturally when we're starving. By consuming these components through coconut oil, we trick the body into inducing autophagy without starving ourselves.

Reishi Mushroom

The Reishi mushroom has been used in Asian traditional medicine for centuries, which determined scientists to study its therapeutic effects. Recent studies suggest that the Reishi mushroom induces autophagy, which can produce anticancer effects in those who suffer from breast cancer.

*** Delicious recipe for Autoph-Tea, one of the easiest ways you can support the activation of autophagy in your cells

- 1 green tea bag

- 1 whole citrus bergamot Earl Grey tea bag

- 1 tablespoon raw coconut oil

- 1 cinnamon stick (Ceylon cinnamon)

- 1 teaspoon monk fruit powder (optional)

In a kettle or small saucepan, bring 1 to 1 ½ cups water to a boil. Pour the water into a large mug and add the tea bags and cinnamon stick. Let steep for at least 3 minutes (the longer the better), then remove and discard the tea bags.

Add the coconut oil and stir it in using the cinnamon stick.

Mix it all together for 20 to 30 seconds. You can also blend the tea to help mix the favors and emulsify the oil.

Take the overwhelm out of reclaiming your health...incorporate small ways like drinking Autoph-Tea daily to yield big results.

Natural Supplements That Boost Autophagy

The following natural supplements can also be used to induce autophagy

Resveratrol

Resveratrol is a compound commonly found in grapes, wine, and soy. This compound induces autophagy that can help inhibit breast cancer cells and can reduce the toxicity within the body.

Nicotinamide

Nicotinamide is a component of the vitamin B complex. Consuming this natural supplement can stimulate the autophagy process, which will reduce the pathologic accumulations that lead to the development of Alzheimer's disease.

Vitamin D

Vitamin D is synthesized naturally by our skin when it's exposed to sunlight. However, not many of us can expose our skin to the sun to produce vitamin D, especially in the cold season. This is why doctors recommend vitamin D supplementation.

Vitamin D can induce a powerful autophagy in the pancreatic cells, which can stimulate the insulin production and help prevent the onset of diabetes.

Melatonin

Melatonin is a hormone that plays an important role in the regulation of our circadian rhythm. Recent studies show that melatonin supplementation can induce autophagy in the brain, protecting it against cell injury. This could prevent several neuropsychiatric conditions.

Ginseng

Ginseng is one of the most popular natural supplements in the world. The ginseng root's active components induce autophagy and they have a protective role against breast cancer cells and melanoma.

The Genetics of Autophagy

Just like every other process in our body, autophagy is controlled directly and indirectly by genes. The genes that control this process determine how efficient it will be in collaborating with the immune system, and how well it will function as we grow older.

The Autophagy On/Off Switch

If autophagy is so efficient in protecting our bodies against harmful agents like bacteria, viruses, and cancer cells, why doesn't it make us immune to them?

Well, unfortunately, the natural autophagy process cannot keep up with the aging process. As our bodies grow older, our cells accumulate more and more debris inside them. The autophagy mechanism is triggered, and the lysosomes start cleaning up the cells. But they simply can't keep up with the workload.

Cells die continuously inside the body. The autophagy process cannot take place continuously in every part of the body. The active process always targets the cells that face the highest stress and works in a maintenance mode everywhere else.

For example, your skin cells face a high stress when you get a sunburn. Some of the cells die and trigger apoptosis, while others are damaged and trigger the autophagy. Sure, your damaged liver cells will still get fixed, but the body's focus is not on them at that moment. It needs to handle the skin burn first. That's the priority.

However, we can activate the autophagy mechanism at will. This can be accomplished in two ways. We can either consume foods or dietary supplements that induce the process, or we can produce some form of stress on the body and trigger it. Fasting and dieting are the easiest and healthiest ways to induce stress as a trigger for autophagy.

The Benefits Of Using Autophagy

As you could see, inducing autophagy presents multiple possible benefits. While this topic is still under scientific scrutiny, most researchers agree that the autophagy process can help us lead better and healthier lives.

1. Autophagy may save your life.

Dramatic? Yes. But, scientifically accurate. Autophagy is an ancient mechanism whose main function is to preserve your life. During times of extreme stress, infection, or starvation, this process kicks in to maximize repair while minimizing damage. The combination of intermittent fasting (with some fat as fuel) while activating autophagy at the same time can both starve an infectious intruder of glucose, reduce inflammation so the immune system has an easier time taking action, and repair damage caused by both infection and inflammation. In short, animals evolved using autophagy to conserve energy and repair damage when energy became scarce, but it is also a critical part of the human immune system's ability to battle illness and reduce risk of cancer.

2. Autophagy may improve your quality and length of life.

Anti-aging benefits may sound too good to be true, but beauty really does run far deeper than the skin. Since the 1950s, scientists have known about the process of autophagy, but recent studies have revealed more about how it improves your cellular health. Instead of taking in new nutrients, cells undergoing autophagy recycle the damaged parts they have, remove toxic material and fix themselves up. When your cells repair themselves, they work better, and they can behave like younger cells. You may have heard or noticed that some people have a very different chronological (time) and biological (life) age. How much toxic damage a body has taken and how it has been able to repair plays a large role in these differences.

3. Autophagy helps your metabolism work better.

Autophagy is a process of taking out trash and replacing cell parts, like mitochondria. Mitochondria are your cellular engines. They burn fat and make ATP, your body's energetic currency.

There is a lot of harsh toxic build up in mitochondria that can damage cells, and breaking them down proactively saves future wear and tear on your cells. Autophagy of other cell parts helps the entire cell work more efficiently not just to burn fuel but also to make proteins. Healthier cells work more efficiently.

4. Autophagy reduces risk of neurodegenerative diseases.

Many diseases of aging brains take so long to develop because they are the result of proteins in and around your brain cells that are misfolded and don't work right. Autophagy helps cells clean up the proteins that aren't doing their jobs and they are less likely to accumulate. For instance, in Alzheimer's disease autophagy removes amyloid, and in Parkinson's autophagy removes α-synuclein. There is a reason dementia is thought of hand-in-hand with diabetes: constant high blood sugar keeps autophagy from activating, making it difficult to keep these cells clear of clutter!

5. Autophagy helps regulate inflammation.

Autophagy promotes a "goldilocks" amount of inflammation by helping to boost or quell the immune response you need. Autophagy can increase inflammation when an invader is present by triggering your immune system to attack. Most of the time, autophagy decreases inflammation from your immune response by removing the signals (proteins called antigens) that are triggering it.

6. Autophagy helps us fight infectious disease.

As mentioned above, autophagy can help recruit an immune response when needed. Secondly, the process of autophagy can remove certain microbes directly from the inside of cells, such as Mycobacterium tuberculosis, or viruses, such as HIV. Autophagy can also remove the toxins created by infections, which is especially important for food-borne illness.

7. Autophagy improves muscle performance.

As you create microtears and inflame muscles during exercise, the muscles require repair. Energy demand increases. Your muscle cells will respond to this by undergoing autophagy to reduce the energy required to use the muscle, degrade damaged components, and improve the balance of energy to reduce the risk of future damage.

8. Autophagy helps prevent cancer onset.

Autophagy can suppress processes that are pro-cancer like chronic inflammation, genome instability, and the DNA damage response. Mice that researchers have genetically engineered to have impaired autophagy have increased rates of cancer. As cancer progresses, it may activate autophagy to get alternative fuel or to hide from the immune system, though more research is needed. It is also unclear how much chemotherapy-induced damage to non-cancerous cells activates autophagy. In the future we may question how much damage chemotherapy does to cancer cells (killing them outright) versus to our own cells (activating autophagy to trigger an immune response that affects these cells). Again, more research is needed.

9. Autophagy improves your digestive health.

The cells that line your gastrointestinal tract are constantly asked to do work. In fact, a large part of your feces are your own cells! As a result of turning on autophagy, your digestive cells can repair and restore, clear themselves of junk, and reduce or activate the immune system as needed. Because a chronic immune response in the gut can overwhelm and inflame your bowels, a chance to rest, repair, and restore is critical to your gut health. Activate autophagy with a schedule that allows for an extended overnight fast and you can give your gut the space it needs to heal.

10. Autophagy improves your skin health.

The cells that you present to the world take a lot of damage from chemicals, air pollution, light, heat, cold, humidity changes, and physical damage. It's a wonder they don't look worse for wear! When your skin cells accumulate damage and toxins, they age in place. Even though you make new cells often, autophagy can help repair the existing ones so that you really glow! Skin cells, in particular, engulf bacteria that may damage the body, so it is very important to support them as they clear out the clutter. Learn more about at-home skin treatments and recipes to support your largest organ in my New York Times bestselling book Glow15 and on my website!

11. Autophagy may support a healthy weight.

Here are some benefits of autophagy that also support a healthy weight:

Autophagy requires fat-burning to be turned on but spares protein. On very long fasts, you will lose protein mass, but in shorter periods of fasting, you can activate autophagy, burn fat, spare protein, and get all the benefits of a leaner, fitter you.

Autophagy quells unnecessary inflammation. Chronic inflammation raises insulin, causing more weight storage– so less inflammation helps reduce insulin levels.

Autophagy reduces toxins in your cells. As long as you can excrete those toxins, they are less likely to need fat cells to store them.

Autophagy supports metabolic efficiency by repairing the parts of cells that make and package proteins and process energy, which is particularly helpful when cells need to switch to fat-burning for energy.

12. Autophagy (cell-eating) minimizes apoptosis (cell death).

Apoptosis is programmed cell death. Compared to autophagy, the death of a cell is messy and creates garbage to clean up. Your body triggers some inflammation to do the clean-up. The more cells that repair themselves before they become damaged beyond repair, the less effort your body puts into cleaning up old cells and making new ones. Less inflammation is involved in renewing tissues. You can use that energy to replace cells that need more constant renewal, like skin or digestive cells. While there are some cells that must be turned over a lot, not all cells require this. More repair with less cleanup is a great combination for success.

While autophagy has many health benefits, it is a repair response to stress and should not be on all the time. In my Glow15 Program, I share with you how to turn autophagy on and off inside your cells to get the best of both worlds!

AUTOPHAGY: THE NEW BIOLOGICAL STRATEGY FOR LONGEVITY

The research on the longevity of living beings is carried out in the field of biogerontology, that sector of biology that deals with knowing the natural mechanisms of aging, mechanisms that determine the life span of organisms (from invertebrates to humans) . Information on these processes (and on the possible possibility of modifying them to slow down the aging process and prolong the existence of individuals) involves a variety of biological disciplines (such as genetics, physiology, biochemistry, general medicine and others) and the results of the studies conducted (which have lasted more than a century generally on animal cells or whole organisms) seem to converge globally on two apparently antithetical general positions: the role of genetic predisposition to aging and the influence of the external environment on lifespan. While in the first case it would be the genes proper to an organism, with their functioning, the main ones responsible for its aging speed (and therefore its long or short duration of existence), in the second perspective to determine the individual differences of longevity would count of plus the lifestyle led by the body (food, disease, pollution, stress, etc.)

Since currently the majority of scholars tend to integrate the two cited proposals (rather than separate), many experts agree that to determine the actual life span of a living being contribute (to varying degrees) both its peculiar genetic component and his way of living (and therefore of eating, doing physical activity, and so on).

The study of the genetic components of longevity is enriched day by day with new information and discoveries (such as those concerning the telomerase enzyme), but it increasingly demonstrates the great complexity of the problem (the high number of genes "in play") , and, to the detriment of the easy hopes of increasing lifespan through pharmacologically targeted genetic manipulations, dangerous (and at the same time not easy to control) side effects emerge (at least for the moment). Therefore, until the roles of all the genes involved in the aging process are known in detail, the interventions aimed at modifying their functioning (for pro-longevity purposes) still appear premature and potentially dangerous.

On the other hand, on the other hand, over half a century of research has shown the prevalence of two fundamental factors capable of increasing life span: physical activity conducted by organisms and the reduction of calories consumed with the daily diet (calorie restriction). Most animal experiments on the effects of physical activity (moderate) agree on the beneficial effect, in terms of health and longevity, of physical exercise: the increase in this activity would result in a lower incidence of metabolic diseases , circulatory and other (in addition to greater longevity) in the subjects who practice it, compared to the more sedentary ones.

Similar results emerge from studies (mainly on rodents and primates) on calorie restriction: animals on a restricted diet of more than 30% of the calories normally taken at meals are significantly healthier and more long-lived than those who eat freely.

If for a long time scientists have not been able to clarify in detail the biological mechanisms underlying these two paradigms, recently in Italy (in Pisa) the research group of Professor Ettore

Bergamini has contributed significantly to unraveling the mystery: the benefits for the health and longevity linked to the reduction of diet calories are intimately linked to a phenomenon inherent in all eukaryotic cells (including ours), that is cellular autophagy. This autophagy, and macroautophagy to be precise, is a phenomenon of recycling and repair of the damaged components of the cell (cytoplasmic proteins, membranes and organelles) due to the incessant harmful action carried out by free radicals (oxidative stress). These radicals, chemically unstable and highly reactive, are substances that are inevitably produced as a result of normal cellular metabolism, inflammation, stress, pollution, etc. and are capable of attacking and seriously damaging the structures of the cell, if not effectively counteracted. itself (like macromolecules and organelles). The latter can avoid succumbing by accelerating its rhythm of division (reproduction), but will thus more quickly reach the condition of senescence (the number of possible divisions is limited) and therefore to premature death. Macroautophagy is thus a rescue system: the oxidized cytoplasmic proteins, the old and damaged organelles (such as the mitochondria, the "energy centers" of the cells) and other important structures are thus isolated from the rest of the cellular cytoplasm and incorporated into said membranous vesicles autophagosomes. Subsequently these autophagosomes fuse into the cytoplasm with lysosomes (organelles full of "digestive" hydrolytic enzymes) which thus pour their content into the autophagosomes themselves and allow the enzymatic demolition (digestion) of the material previously sequestered there. In this way, the cells can, for example, degrade damaged proteins (autophagic proteolysis) by then recycling many "building materials" (amino acids) for energy or reconstruction purposes. These cells, therefore, having repaired the damage and being renewed in their fundamental structures, can slow down the rhythm of division and therefore live longer. Macroautophagy is normally mildly induced during the first 24 hours of fasting (a form of short-term caloric restriction) of animals (laboratory rats) mainly in the internal organs (such as the liver), but is totally suppressed in the period immediately following at meals. The Bergamini team has discovered that autophagy tends, however, to naturally weaken as animals age (perhaps due to the progressive inevitable accumulation of oxidative stress damage), but it can be significantly intensified even in older animals through the use (coupled with fasting) of particular drugs called anti-hypolithic drugs, capable of blocking the release of fat in the blood (for energy purposes) from adipose tissue. Pharmacologically treated rodents in this way were much less subject to age-related diseases (cardio-vascular problems, diabetes, tumors) than untreated animals of the same age that continued to feed at will (the controls). The first experiments with the method also started on human volunteers and, according to Bergamini himself, show very encouraging results.

hormone insulin (a pathological characteristic present in many elderly people), a precursor to diabetes and, in general, to cellular aging.

In essence, science is now able to fully re-evaluate ancient health precepts (a brief, occasional fast and frequent and moderate physical activity) to be performed at any age and to be used, for preventive purposes, from an early age, to try to stay in health and to slow aging, at least in part.

Cell death: difference between necrosis, apoptosis and autophagy

Cell death can be implemented in various ways and for different causes (physiological or pathological).

Apoptosis

Apoptosis is a type of programmed cell death that occurs physiologically and / or pathologically in response to different stimuli: physiological stimuli for apoptosis can occur in:

selection of cells in tissues in active proliferation (for example, selection of lymphocytes that respond to self in the bone marrow)

cell selection during embryogenesis

elimination of cells that are no longer useful (such as lymphocytes after the removal of an antigen).

Pathological stimuli that induce apoptosis are generally due to: DNA damage (unrepairable), abnormal folding of proteins, infections. The activation of apoptosis can occur through two pathways that converge on the same effector proteins (caspases). The most common way is called intrinsic or mitochondrial because it is mediated by these organelles: the control of apoptosis is guaranteed by the balance of the anti- and pro-apoptotic signals by proteins called BCL. These form channels on the mitochondrial surface that regulate their permeability: the main antiapoptotic factor is BCL2, while the most important proapoptotic BCLs are BAX and BAK. In reality these molecules act by dimerization and the prevalence of dimers leads to the apoptotic cell. If the action of BCL2 prevails over the others, the cell does not undergo apoptosis but if proteins called BH3only sensors of cellular stress intervene, the BAX and BAK channels open and let out the mitochondria proapoptotic enzymes that activate the caspases (for example the cytochrome c). the caspase activated in the intrinsic pathway is caspase 9 while caspases 8 and 10 are involved in the extrinsic pathway (of which the effector caspase is 3); the latter begins with binding to specific receptors on the cell membrane of death signals including TNFa, TNFb, FADD and FAS. The link between FAS and its ligand (FASL / CD95) is a coreceptor in the link between cytotoxic T lymphocytes and the corresponding APC. The interaction between these death signals and their receptors activate the intracellular procaspases 8 and 10 and the effector phase begins.

This involves the activation by the caspases of endonucleases that break the DNA and the degradation of the cytoskeleton by the caspases themselves. The residues of the dead cell form the so-called apoptotic bodies that are phagocytosed because they express molecules (usually intracellular) on the membrane that are recognized by macrophages.

Necrosis

Necrosis occurs only in pathological conditions when cellular damage is not reversible. Under conditions of hypoxia or even of ischemia (which causes more serious damage because the cell is also deficient in nutrients due to anerobic metabolism), the reduction of oxidative phosphorylation leads to a depletion of ATP and a consequent malfunction of the sodium-potassium-ATP dependent pump. Since the transit of ions into and out of the cell is compromised, the cell itself and the organelles increase their size due to osmotic swelling; not only: the incoming $Ca2+$ is increased and this determines the activation of different enzymes that degrade both the DNA and the cellular membrane which at this point disintegrates forming myelinated figures typical of necrosis and causing cell rupture. The release of intracellular enzymes can lead to damage to the surrounding tissue.

Various types of necrosis can be distinguished based on the morphology of the damaged tissue: coagulative necrosis, colliquative, fibrinoid, caseosa, gangrenous, steatonecrosis.

Coagulative necrosis is a type of necrosis generally resulting from ischemic damage due to obstruction of a vessel; in this type of necrosis the architecture of the tissue is generally preserved (in the first days, after which the cellular debris is phagocytized) because there is the denaturation of proteolytic enzymes which therefore cannot fulfill their function of degradation of structural proteins. An area of coagulative necrosis (following ischemia) is called infarction.

Colliquative necrosis is typical of the outbreak of bacterial infection and ischemia of the brain. Necrotic tissue is liquid and viscous because cellular debris is digested. The presence of dead leukocytes in the necrotic tissue gives it a yellowish color, in this case the liquid is called pus.

Gangrenous necrosis refers mainly to the limbs that present a blood supply deficit (and therefore a picture of coagulative necrosis). If the gangrene of the limbs overlaps a bacterial infection, the necrosis assumes the characteristics of a colliquative form for which one speaks of wet gangrene.

Caseous necrosis owes its name to the whitish appearance and the fragile consistency of the necrotic tissue; it is typical of the tuberculosis infection in which there is the formation (above all at the pulmonary level) of a complex with a central necrotic area surrounded by giant Langhans cells (macrophages morphologically transformed into epithelioid cells merge to form giant cells) and lymphocytes, called granuloma.

Steatonecrosis indicates areas of adipocyte necrosis often due to secretion of pancreatic lipases in the organ or peritoneal cavity (acute pancreatitis). The fat cells break and the triglycerides that release the fatty acids escape, which react with calcium forming whitish deposits visible in the organ concerned with a process called fat saponification.

Fibrinoid necrosis is typical of type III hypersensitivity reactions (mediated by immune complexes) in which the deposition and accumulation of antigen-antibody complexes and fibrous tissue inflames and damages the vessel walls, forming a pink-colored thickening around the clearly visible vessel under the microscope.

Autophagy

Autophagy is a process that the cell generally puts into practice in the event of nutrient deficiency; provides phagocytosis of its own organelles that are included in autophagic vacuoles that merge with lysosomes. Defective organelles and proteins are sequestered in double-membrane vesicles, autophagosomes:

induction: it is regulated by mTOR, a kinase that acts as a sensor of available energy levels and amino acids.

autophagosome formation: cytoplasmic material of various nature is incorporated into the autophagosome thanks to enzymes

recognition and fusion of the lysosome autophagosome: ensured, by different proteins including SNARE (membrane proteins that favor the attachment of vesicles);

demolition of the autophagic body: the content of the autophagolisosome is degraded by lysosomal hydrolases.